Dedication

For J,
who shows us every day what real strength looks like.

And for all kids with diabetes—
we see you,
we believe in you,
and we are proud of you.

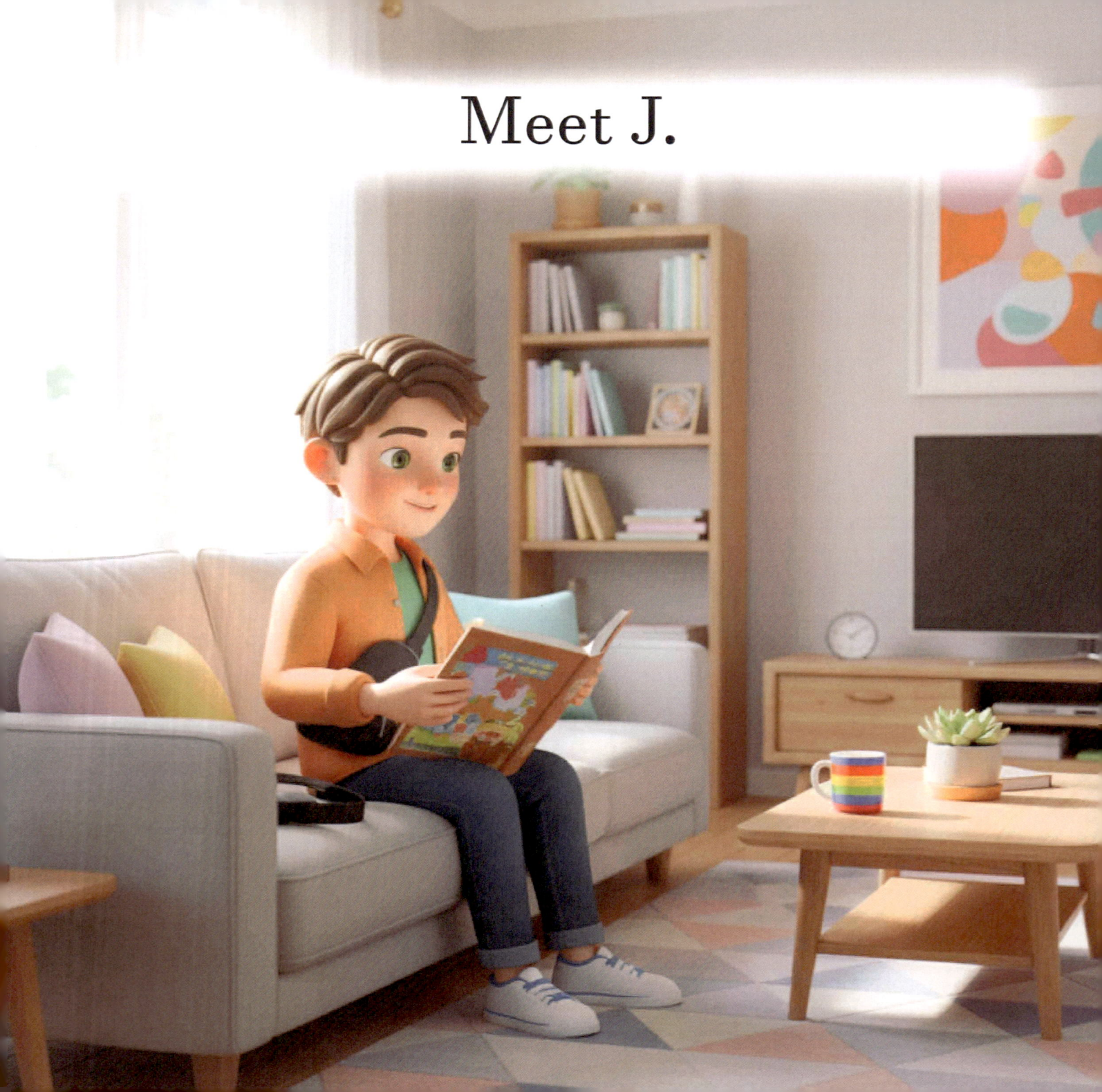
Meet J.

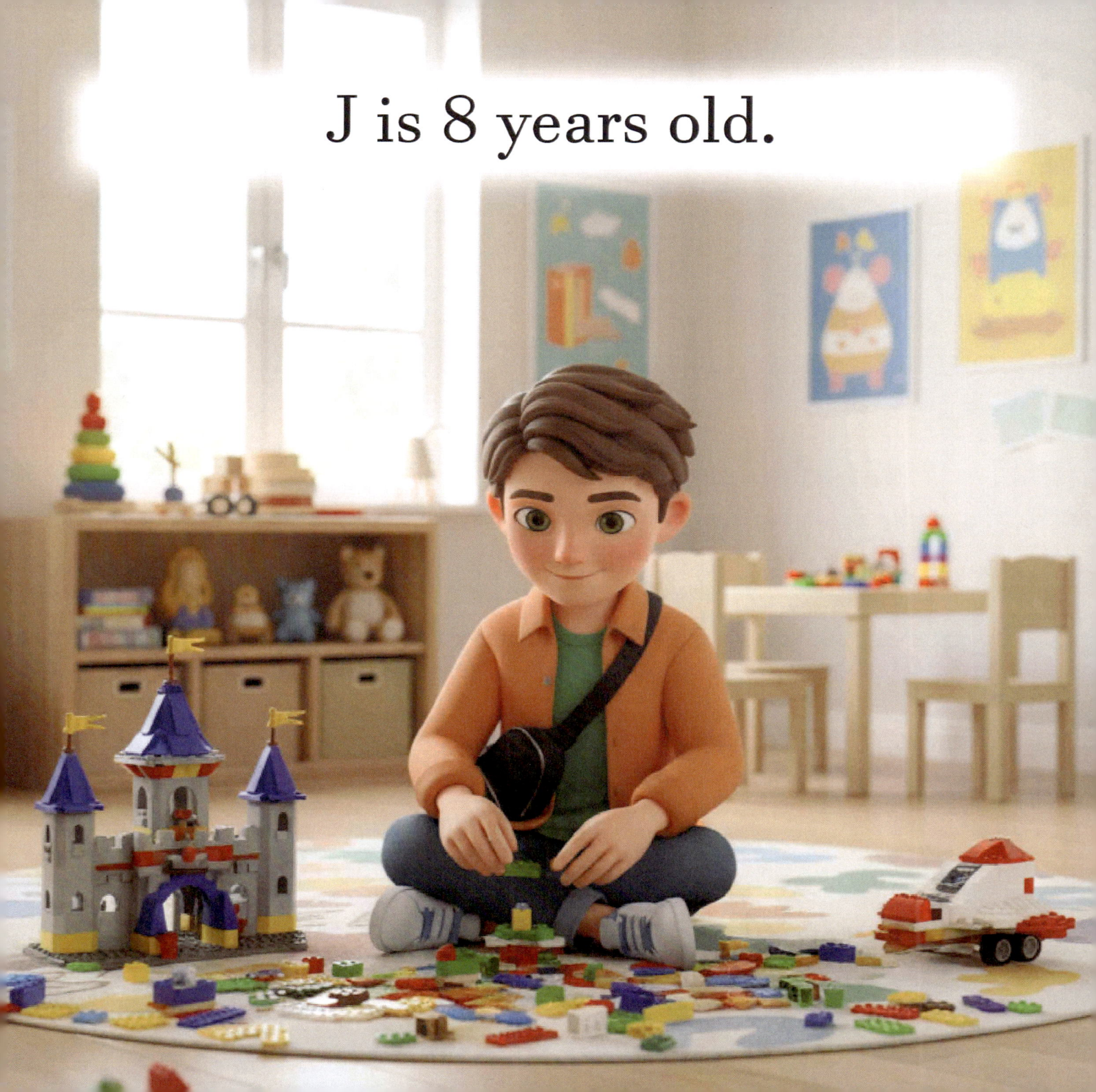

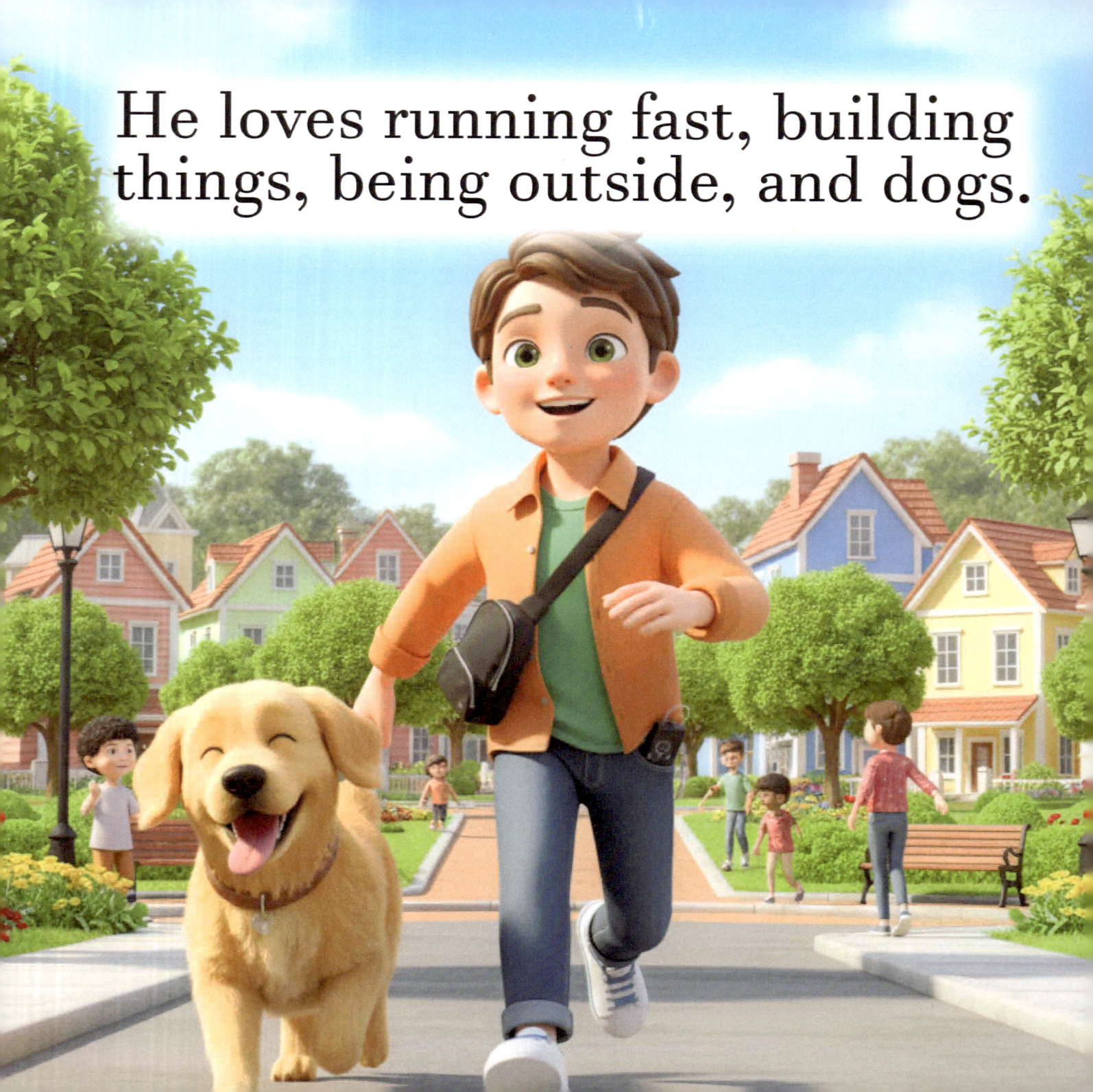

He loves running fast, building things, being outside, and dogs.

J is just like other kids.

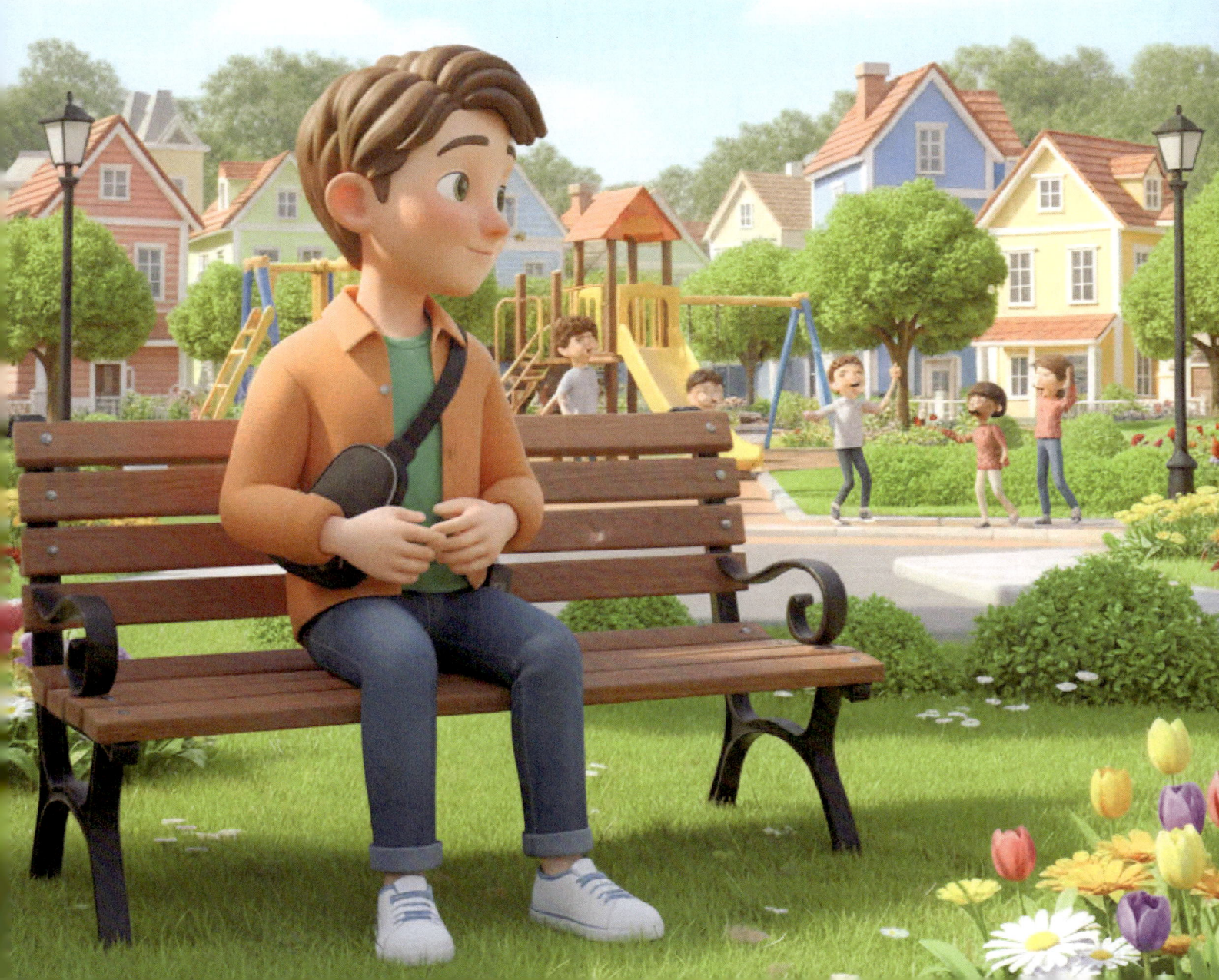

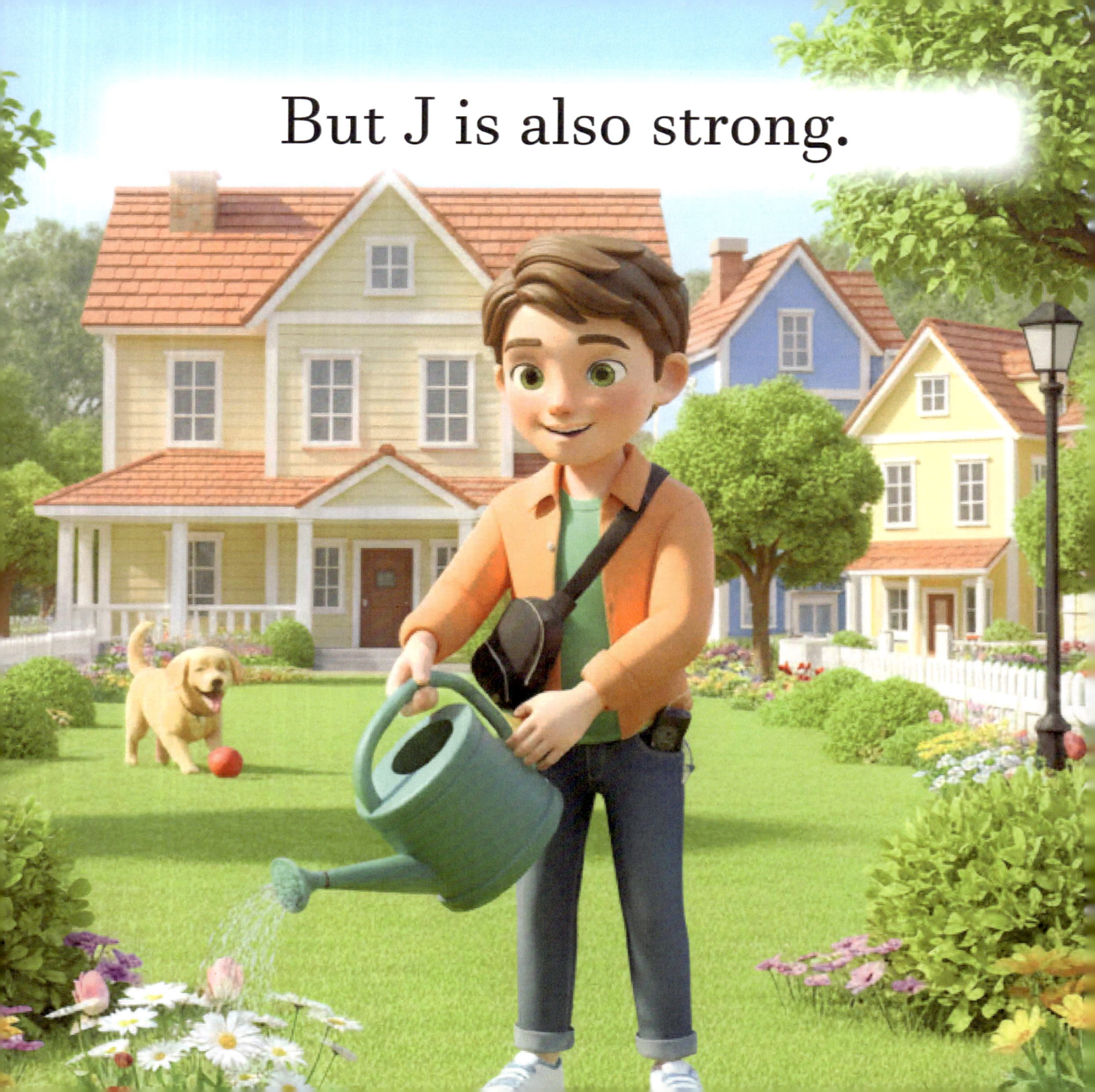
But J is also strong.

J has Type 1 Diabetes.

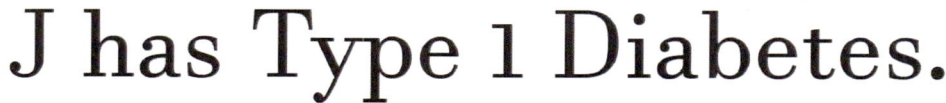

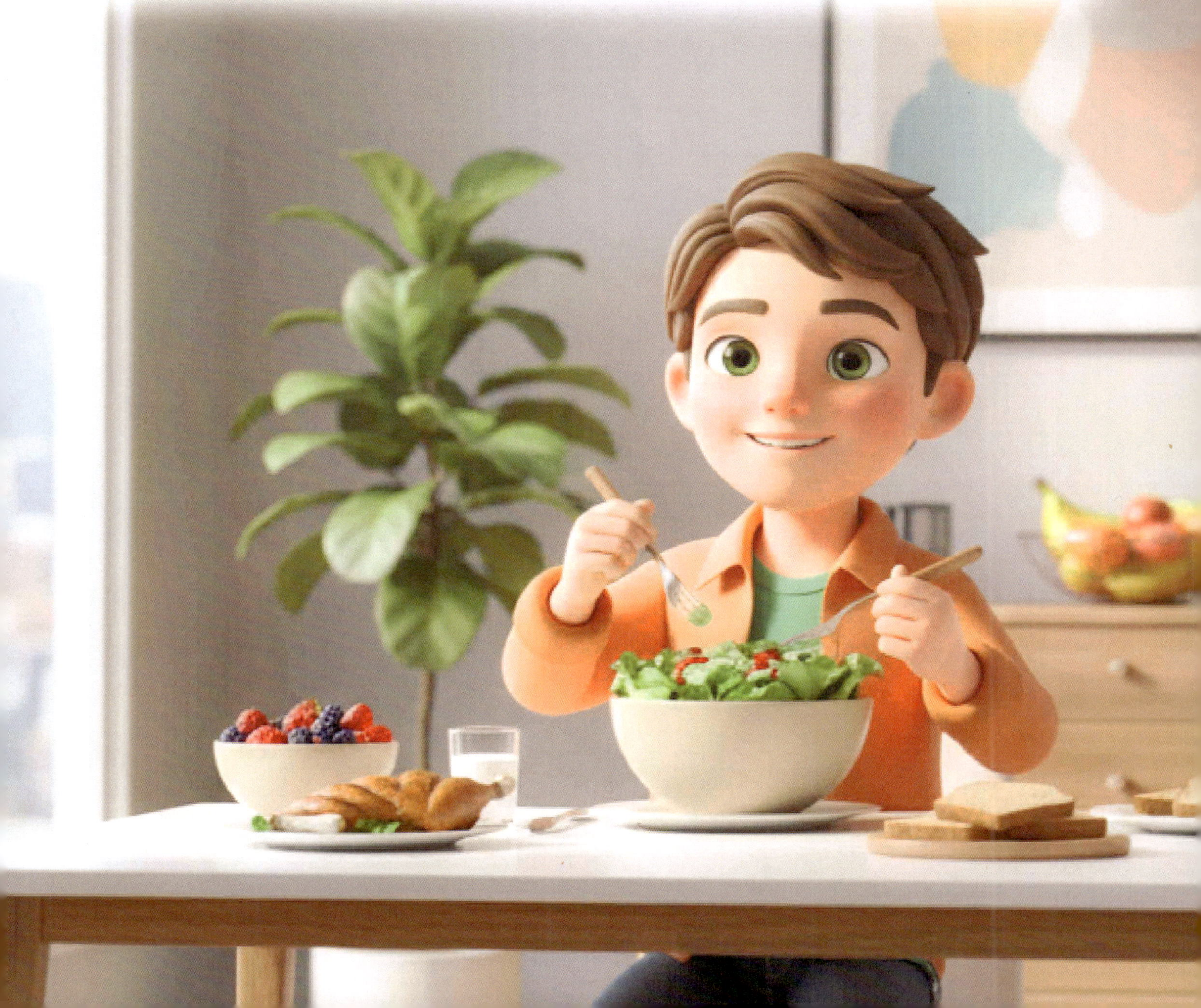

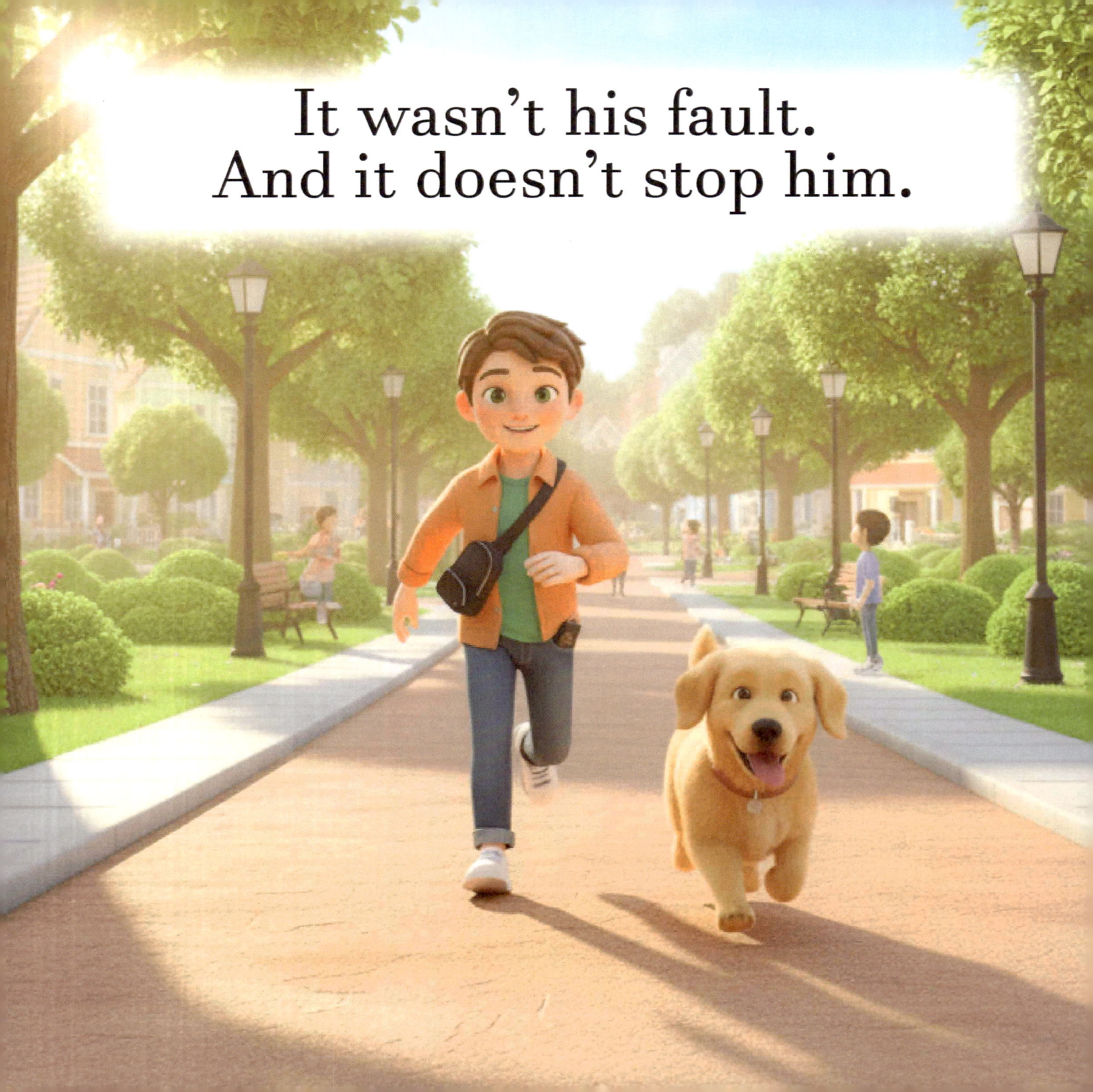
It wasn't his fault.
And it doesn't stop him.

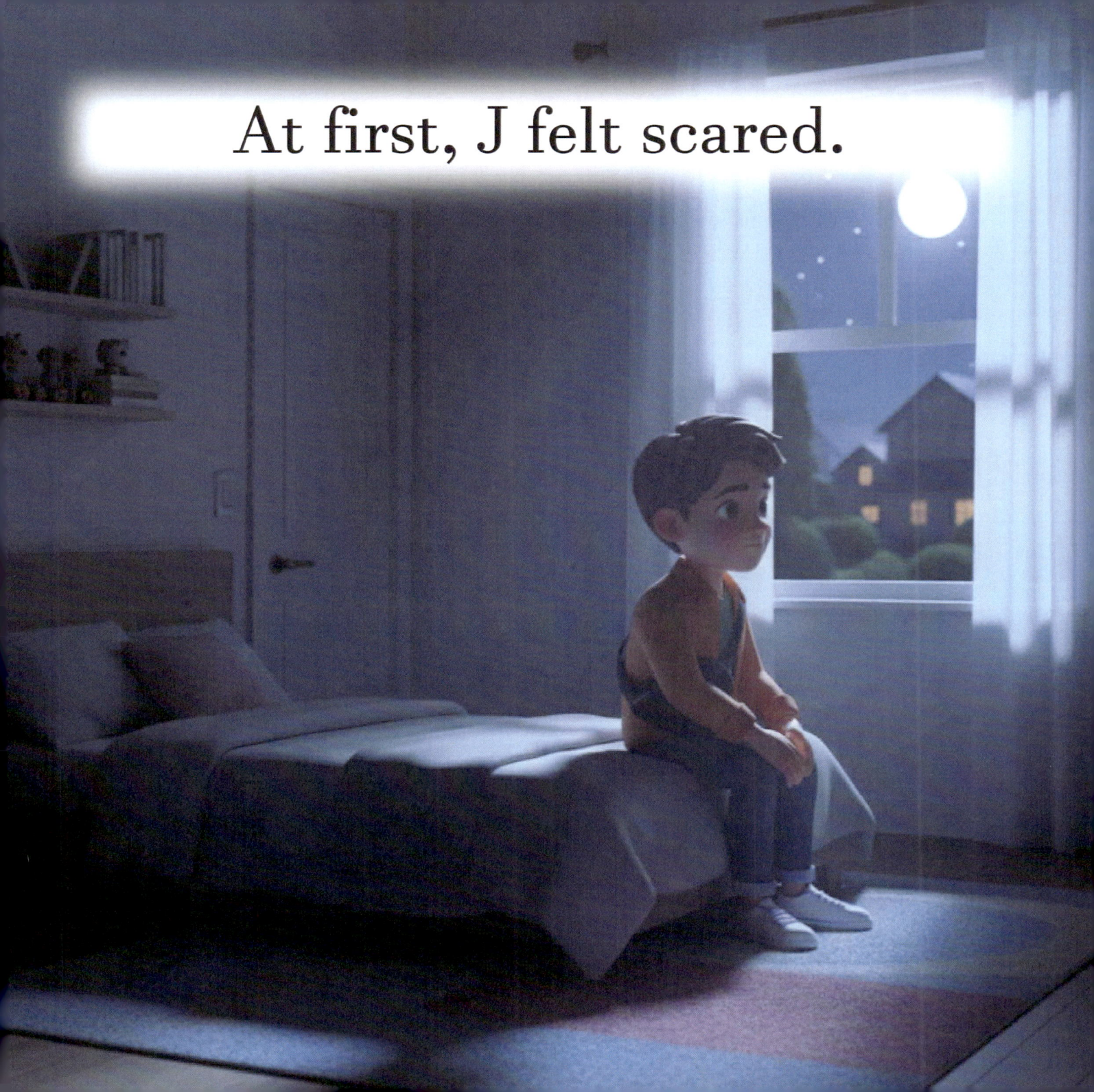
At first, J felt scared.

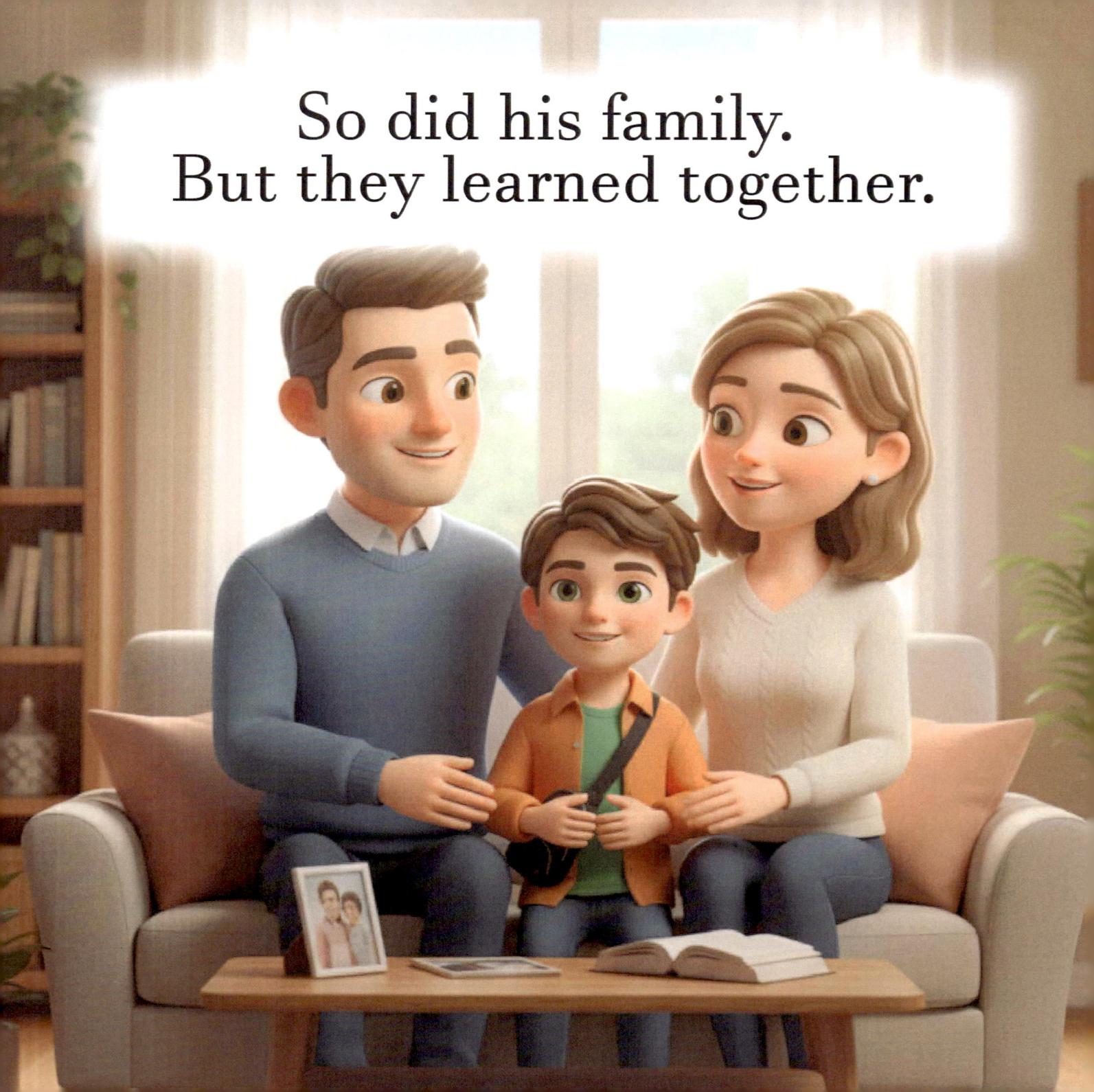

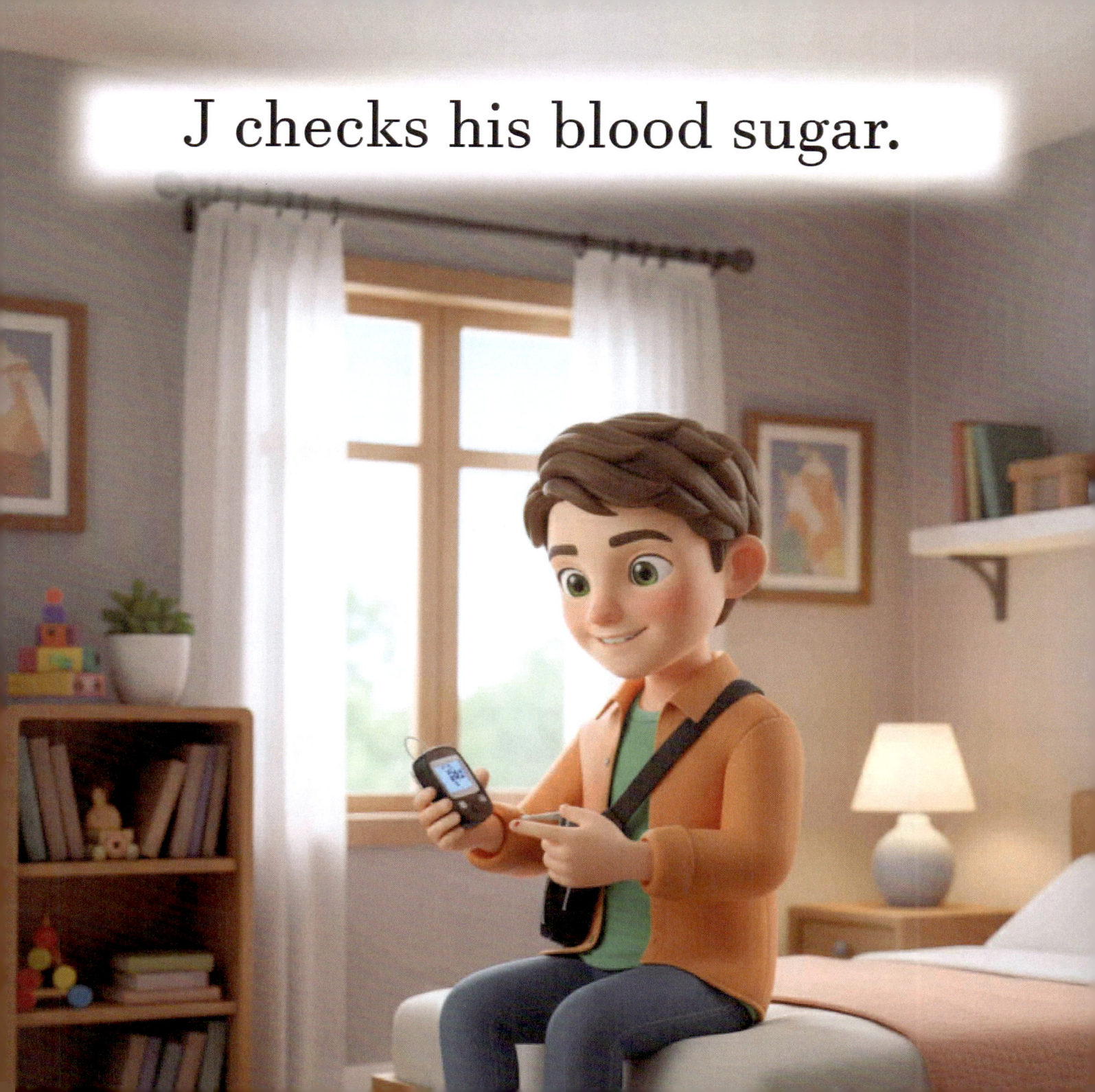
J checks his blood sugar.

J takes insulin.
Strong means doing hard things.

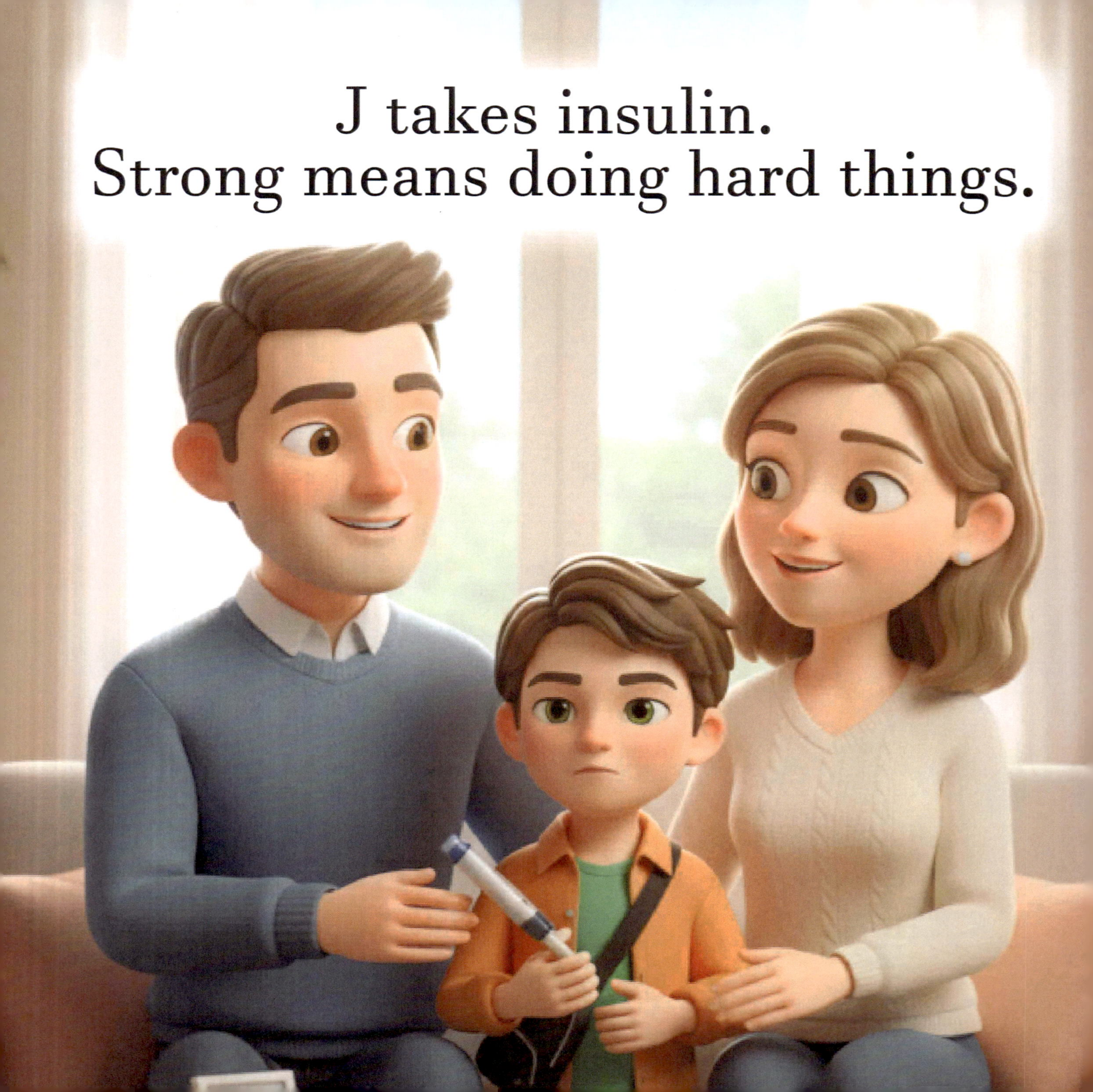

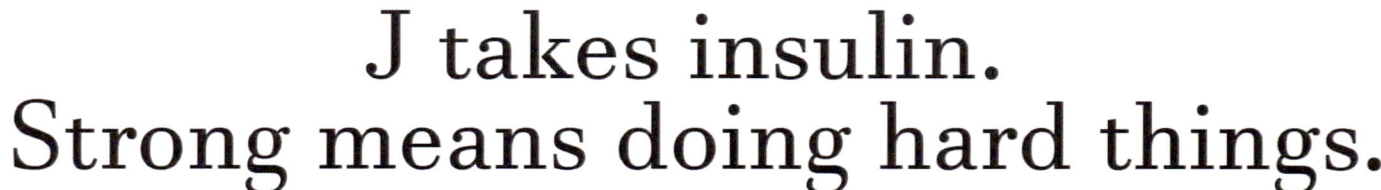

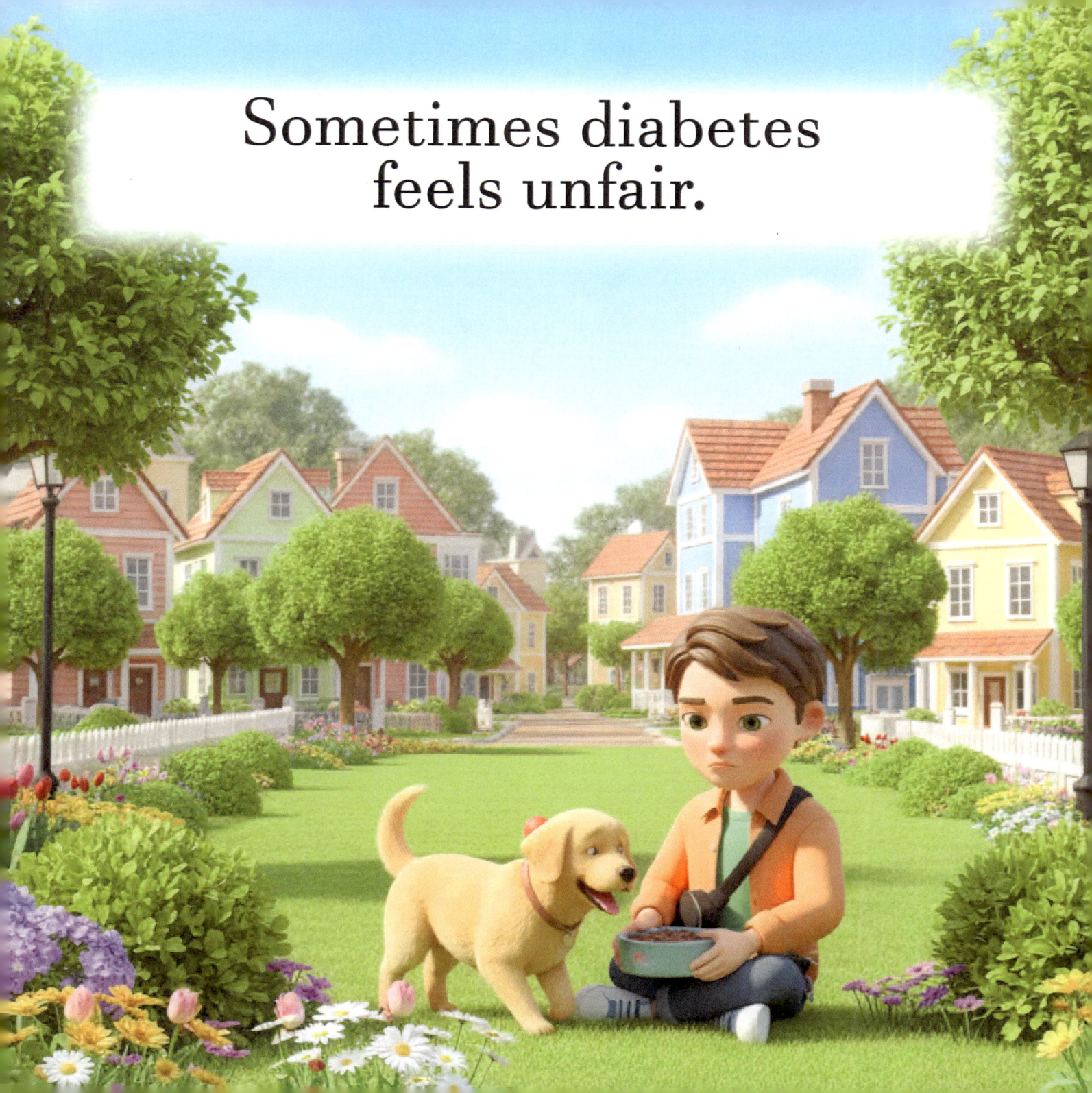

Sometimes diabetes feels unfair.

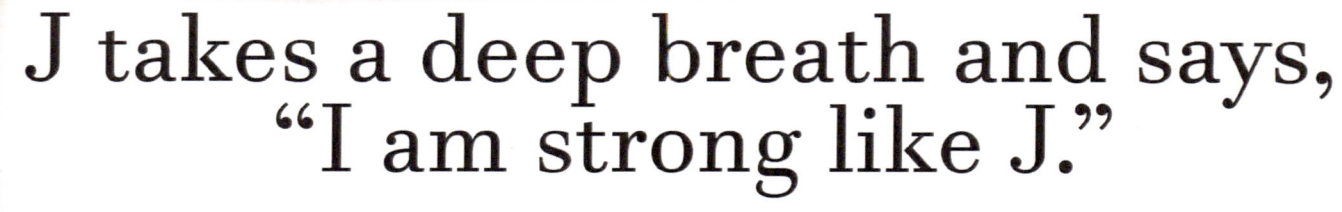

J takes a deep breath and says, "I am strong like J."

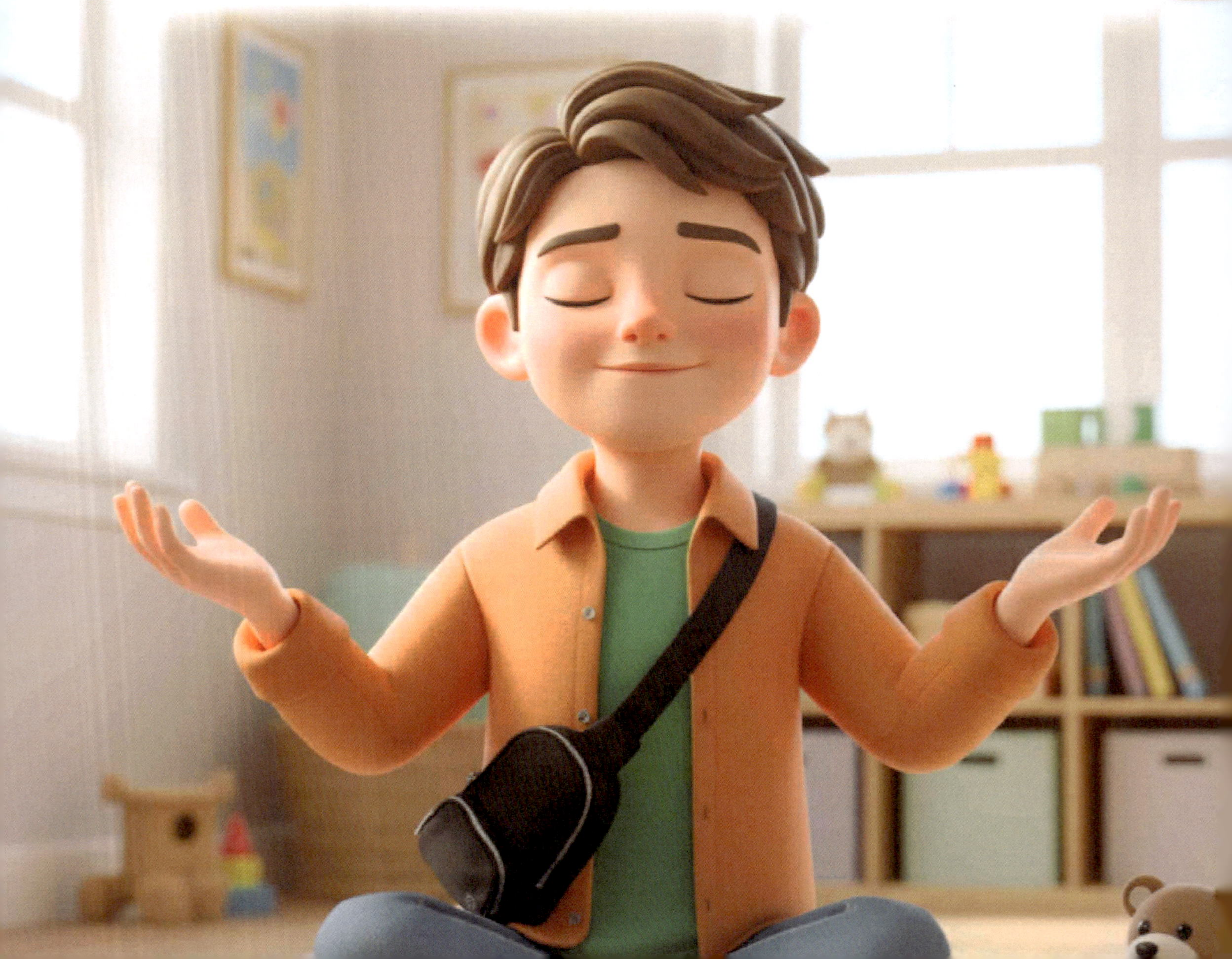

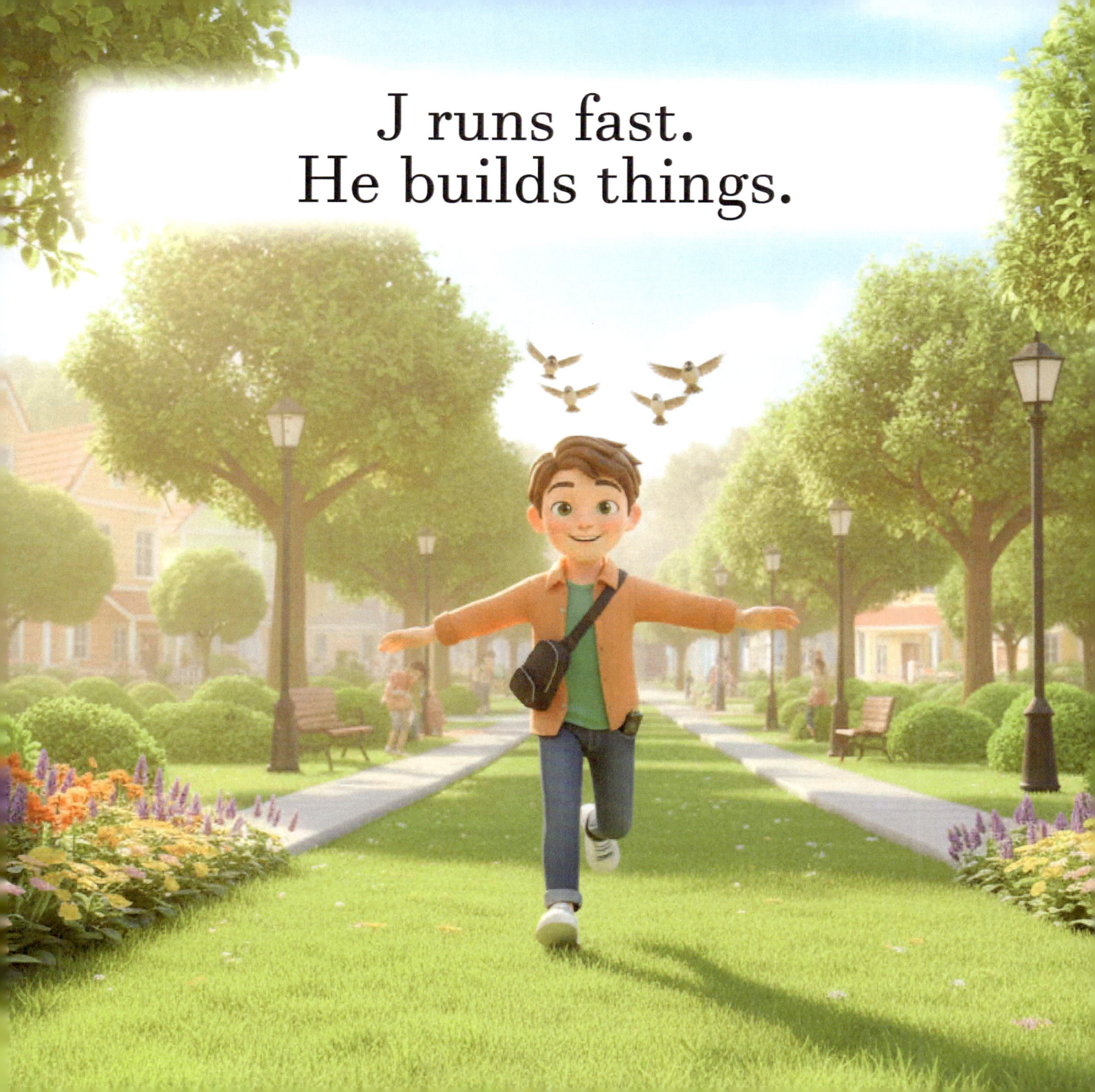
J runs fast.
He builds things.

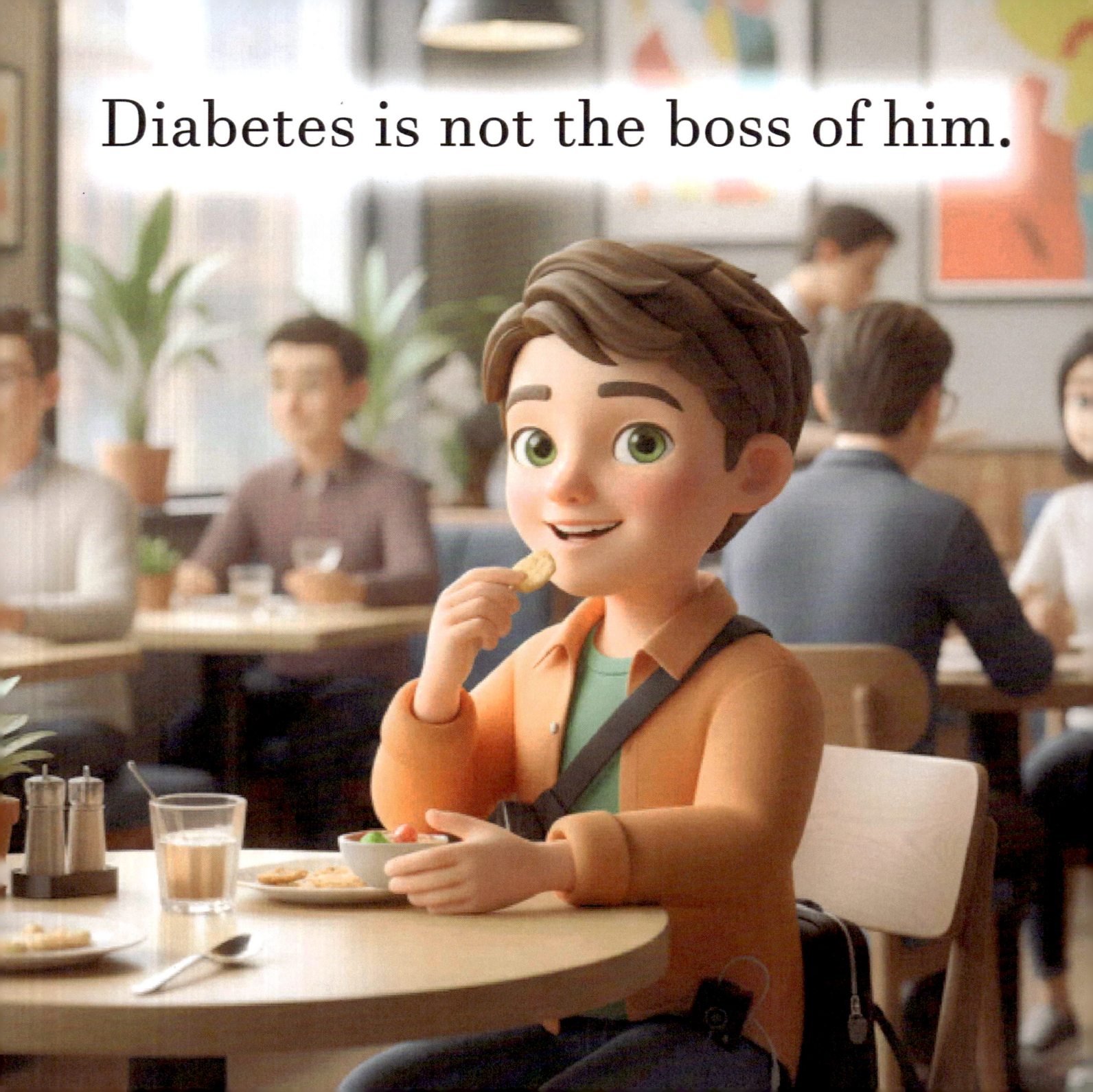
Diabetes is not the boss of him.

One day, J learned about Diabetic Alert Dogs.

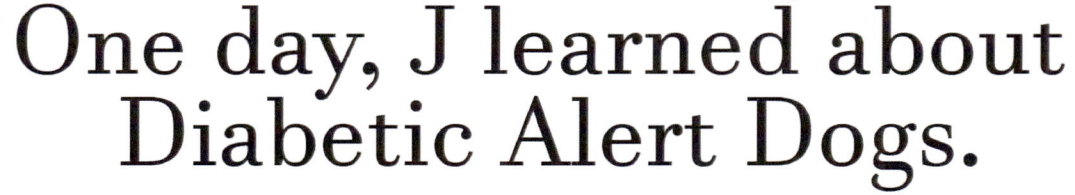

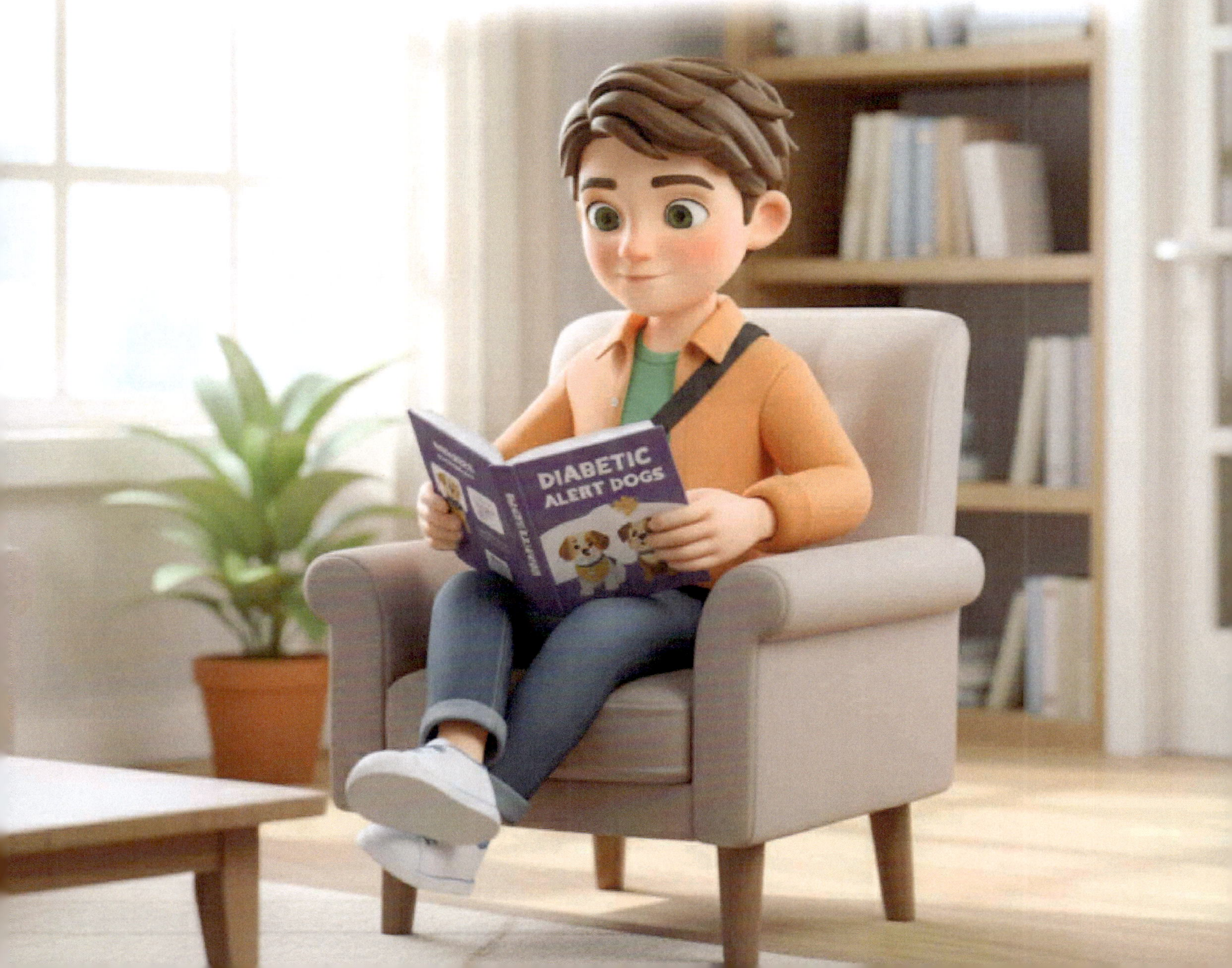

These dogs can smell blood sugar changes and help keep kids safe.

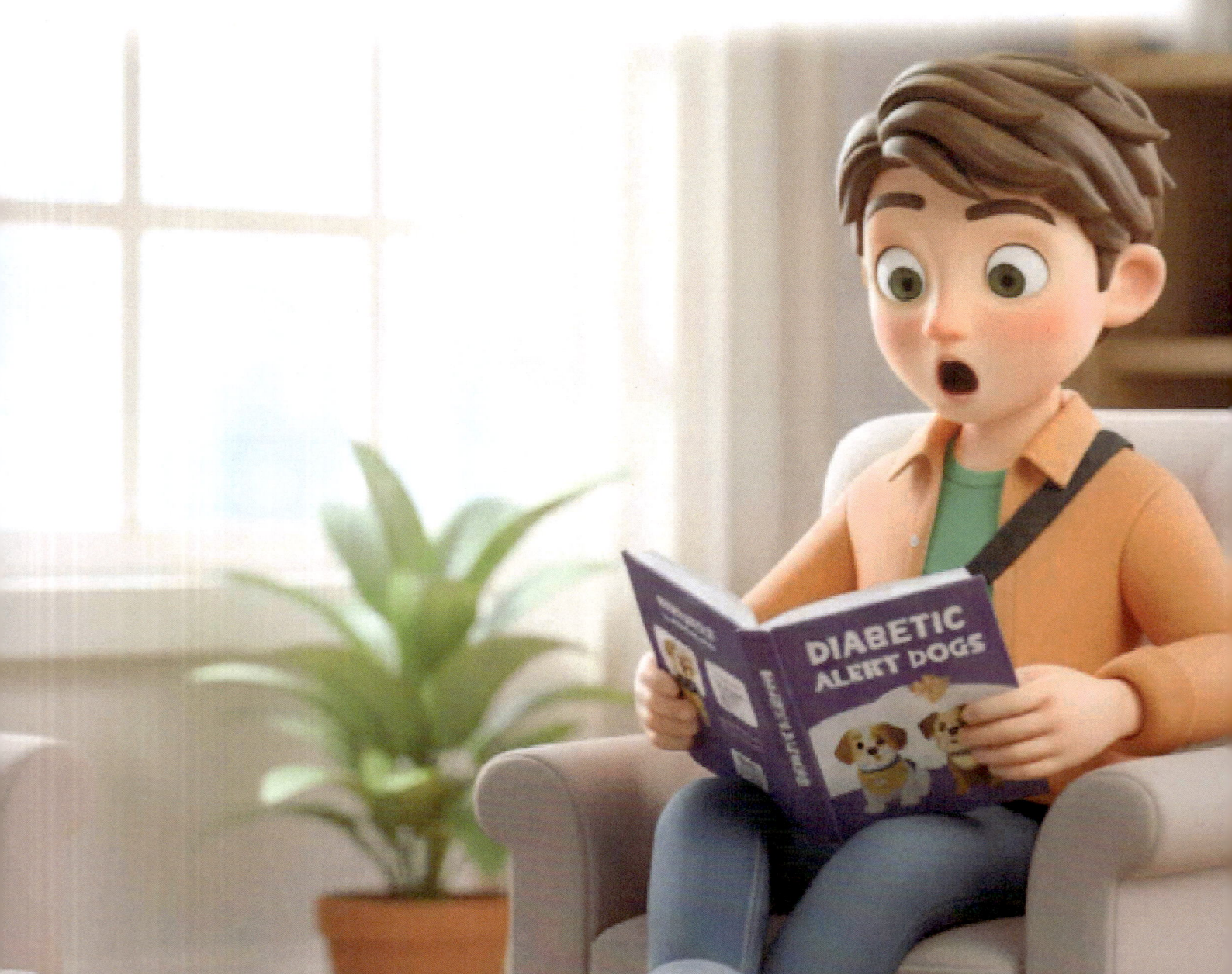

J dreams of a dog by his side.

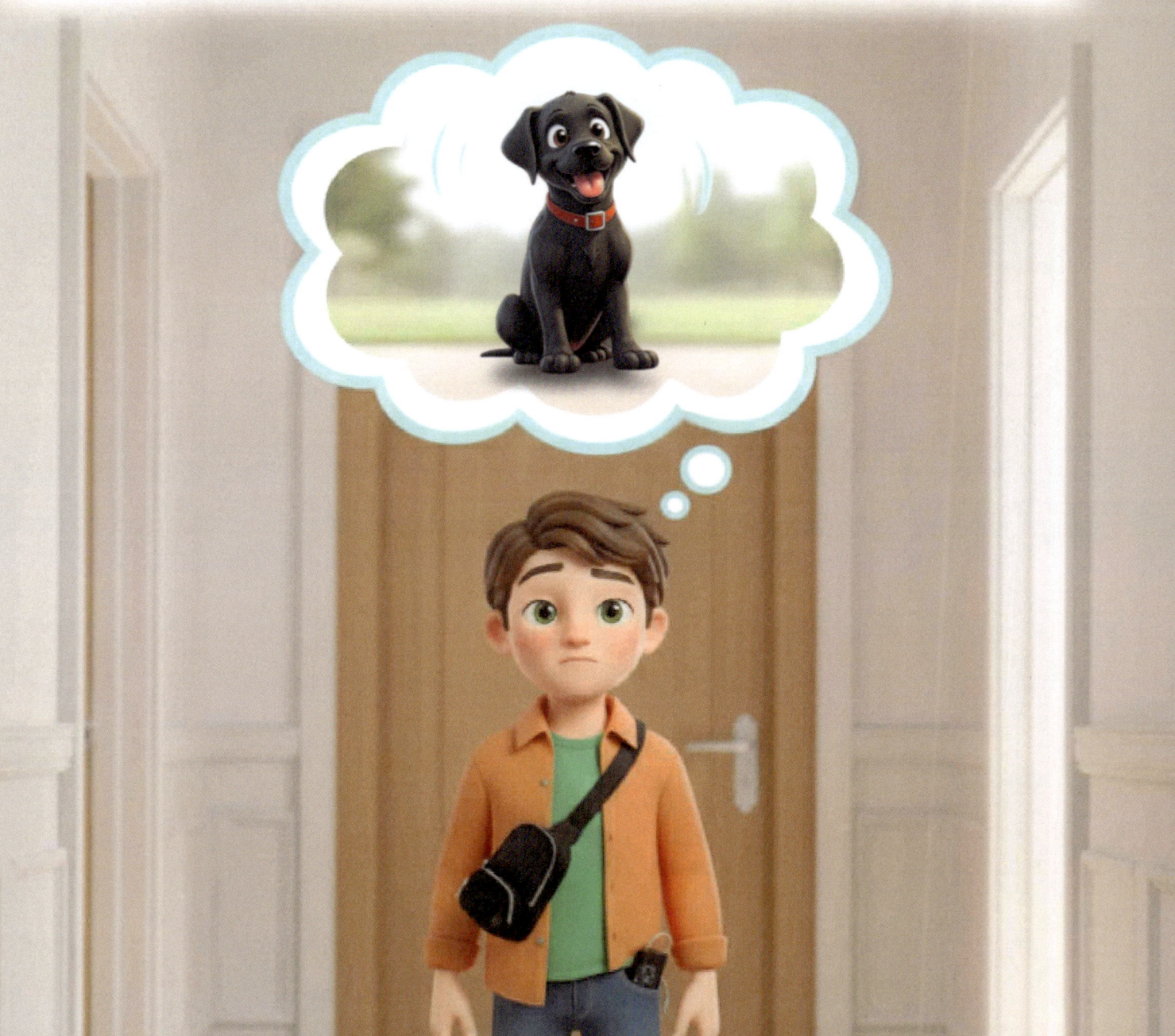

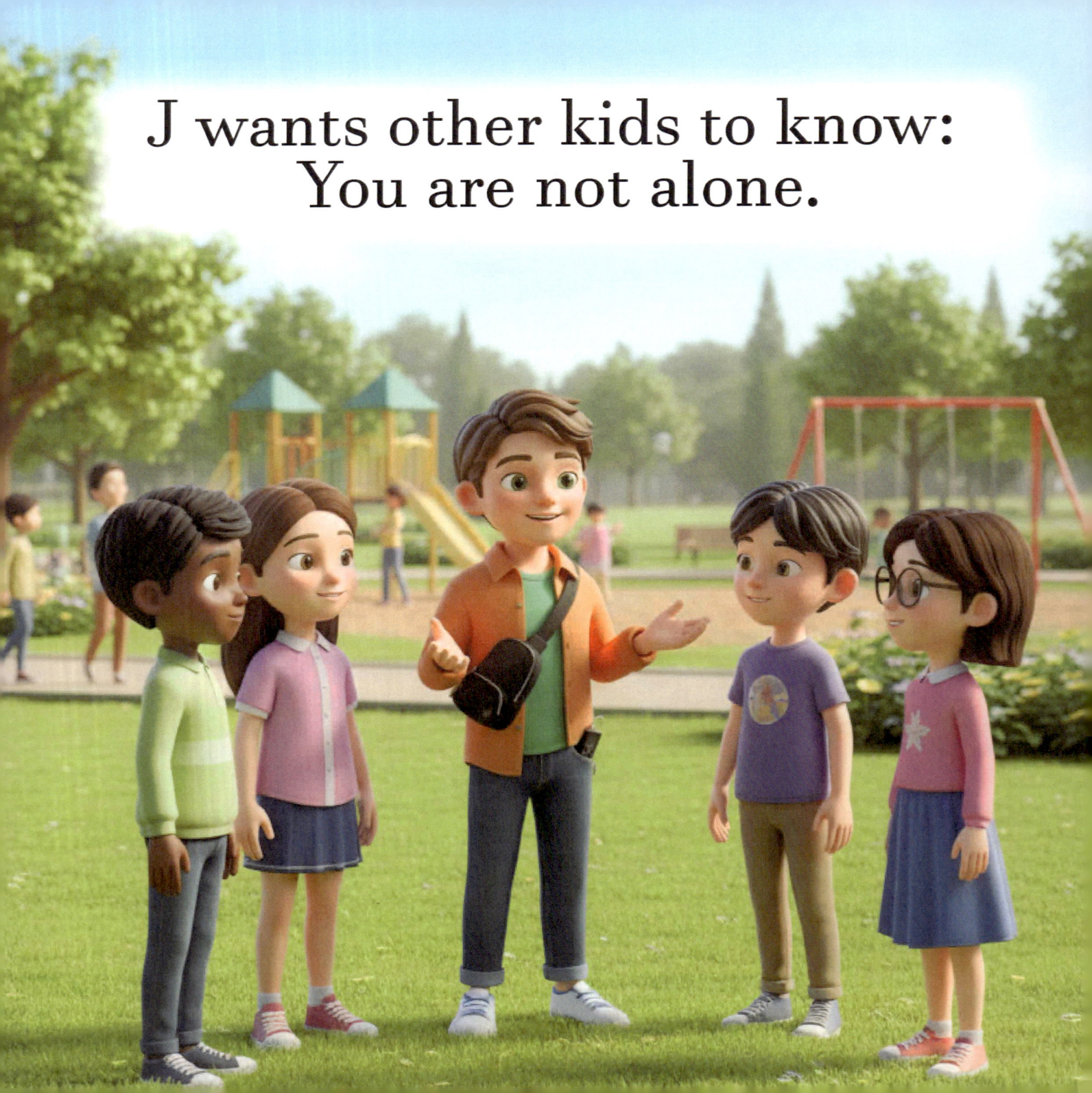
J wants other kids to know: You are not alone.

You are strong too.

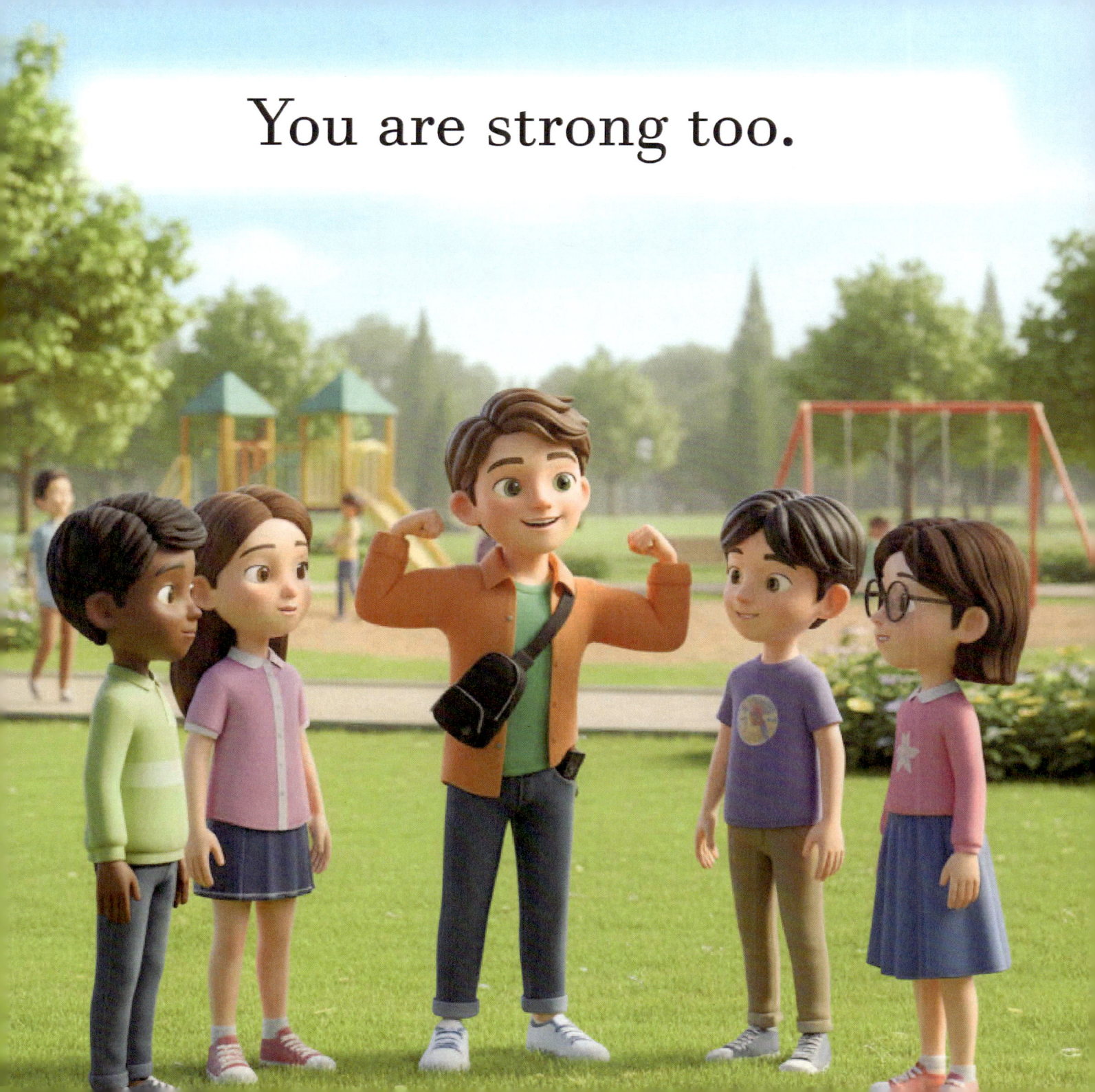

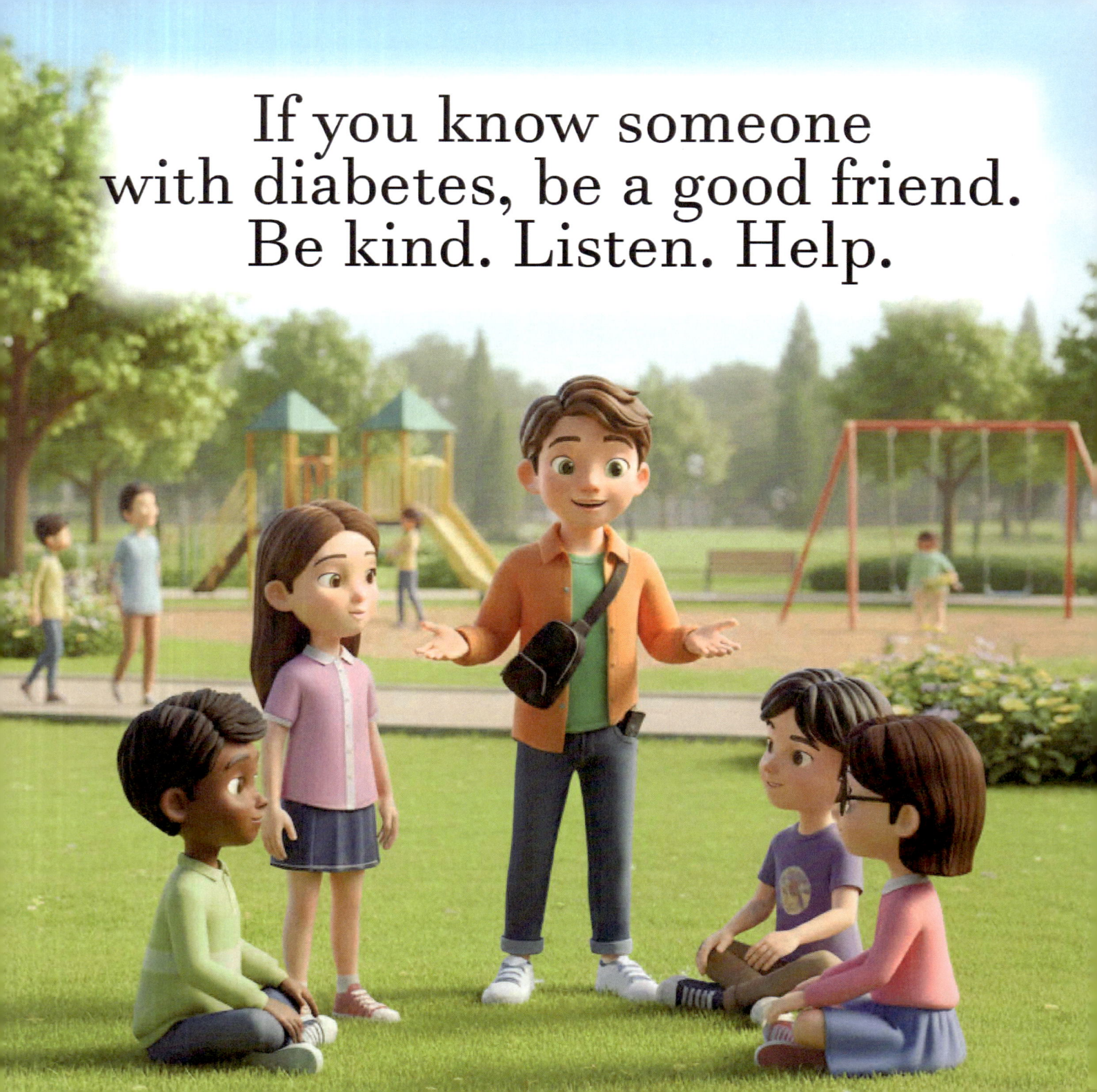

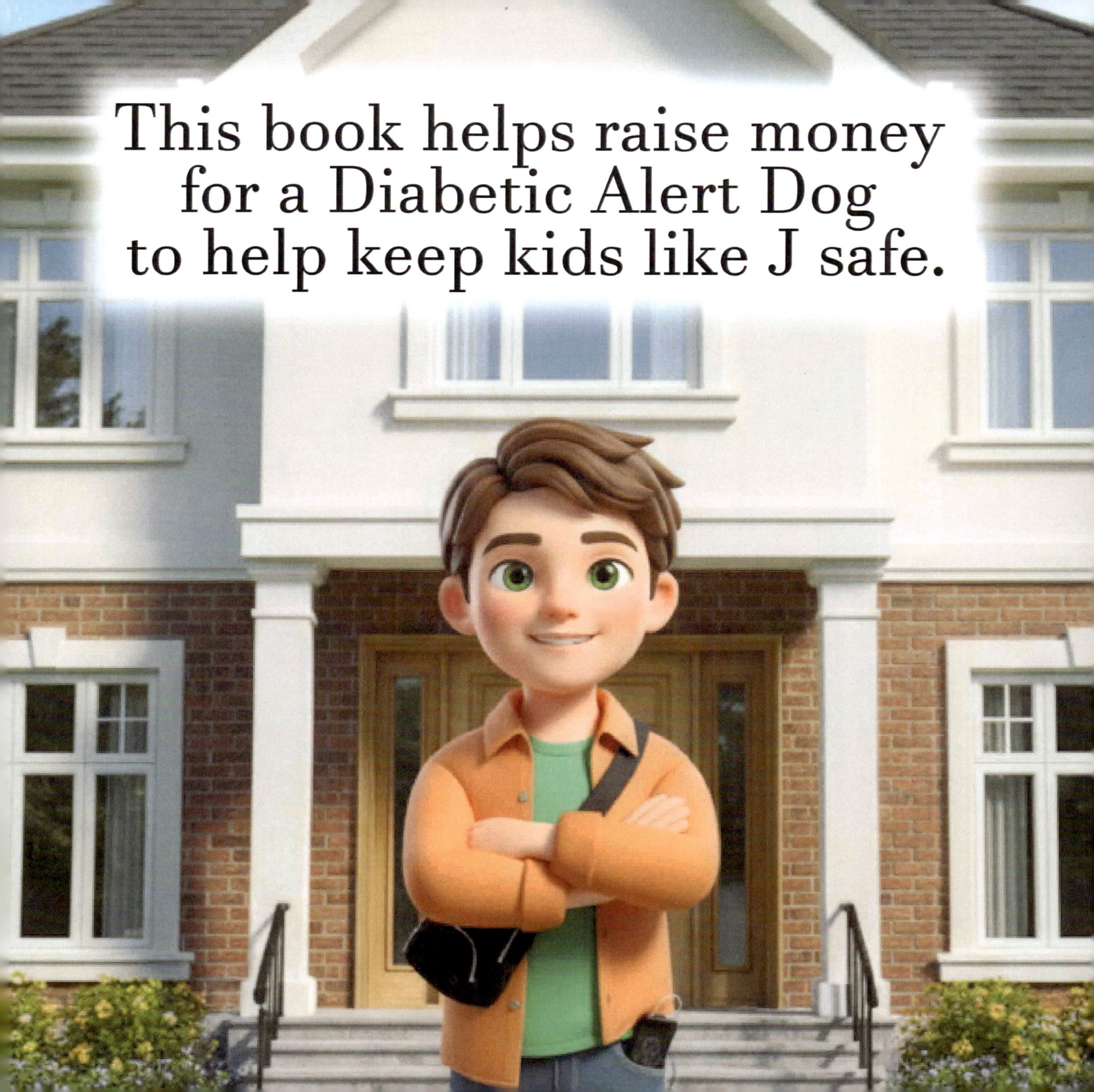

This book helps raise money for a Diabetic Alert Dog to help keep kids like J safe.

The End

Be strong.
Be brave.
Be strong like J.

www.ingramcontent.com/pod-product-compliance
Lightning Source LLC
Chambersburg PA
CBRC101144030426
42337CB00009B/71